THE ULTIMATE
WALL PILATES
WORKOUT GUIDE
FOR BEGINNERS

PROVEN & EASY TO FOLLOW WALL PILATES EXERCISES TO TRANSFORM
YOUR BODY, BURN FAT & FEEL GREAT.

21 DAY ACTION PLAN

JOHN WILLIAMSON

TABLE OF CONTENTS

FUNDAMENTALS OF WALL PILATES FOR A STRONGER AND LEANER YOU

There are many kinds of exercises out there, but wall Pilates is a particularly great option for many individuals who want to give their bodies a boost without any risk of injuring themselves. It's safe, easy, fun, and can easily be tailored to your current fitness levels, which is one of the reasons it has become so popular in recent years.

If you're looking to build up your muscles and tone your body so you enjoy a lean appearance, wall Pilates could be a great option for you. Let's look at both of these areas!

STRENGTH

Firstly, strength. Wall Pilates is an effective way to build up muscle strength for a number of reasons. One of the most important is that it targets lots of muscles that other forms of exercise don't, meaning that you'll build up strength in areas that may be significantly weaker and more difficult to train. Wall Pilates is ideal for targeting muscle groups such as your inner thighs, your internal obliques, y

our iliopsoas, and your stabiliser muscles. Some of the muscles that tend to be exercised by wall Pilates exercises are the ones that are the hardest to target with conventional exercises, so don't underestimate the value of this kind of exercise – even if you also do other kinds of exercise. Wall Pilates is an excellent complement to many forms of working out.

One of the biggest benefits of building up your strength in this way is that it is low impact. There is minimal risk of injuring yourself, pulling or straining muscles, or causing other problems as a result of undertaking wall Pilates, making it an excellent choice for individuals everywhere.

Pilates is particularly known for its ability to enhance your core and we'll look at this in more detail later – but it's unquestionably a great way to build up your muscle strength throughout your whole body.

Lean Muscles

As you start to use and exercise your muscles, you will notice them becoming bulkier – but Pilates is great for creating a lovely leanness in your body. It doesn't bunch the muscles up, but instead encourages them to lengthen and expand.

This can make them look leaner, improving your overall physique and potentially making you feel more confident. If you want to achieve a sleek appearance with trim, long muscles, wall Pilates is a great exercise to try.

Of course, no exercise will make you noticeably taller or give you longer limbs, but wall Pilates will target the muscles in ways that enhance their leanness, rather than bulking them up and making them heavier. This can help you to look taller.

A lot of people feel that Pilates really benefits their bodies, giving them a better range of motion and more capacity to stretch. If you are seeking that sort of result, you'll probably love how wall Pilates makes your body feel.

One of the things that makes Pilates particularly beneficial is that it can be easily adapted to suit an individual's needs. Whether you are already an experienced athlete looking to train your core, somebody who is suffering from an injury and trying to rehabilitate their body, an elderly person looking for exercises that are safe and helpful, or anybody else, wall Pilates can be tailored to help you feel stronger, without putting you at risk of injuries.

Next, we're going to look at how wall Pilates can help you lose weight – which will further enhance the lean look you're aiming for!

THE BENEFITS OF WALL PILATES
FOR WEIGHT LOSS

Of course, one of the top things many people consider when it comes to starting a new exercise regime is how much weight they are likely to lose and how quickly. This isn't of critical importance to everyone, but it's relatively likely to be a consideration.

Wall Pilates may not be the top kind of exercise for losing weight, but it can certainly still help, and it's a key exercise option for many individuals who cannot undertake high-impact workouts.

A good wall Pilates exercise regime can burn a surprising number of calories, and a lot of individuals find this kind of exercising more enjoyable, which means that they are more likely to stick at it in the long term.

This is the best way to create sustainable weight loss, because you will see lasting results if you successfully make exercise a standard part of your routine.

Wall Pilates isn't the ultimate option for losing weight, but it's still a good choice to make, and you will be doing a full-body workout in most cases. This is one of its major benefits; you may not finish your workout sessions drenched in sweat, but you will be using your whole body to burn calories, and you'll lose weight as a result.

It's also very important to note that doing Pilates regularly can increase your basal metabolic rate. This is the rate at which your body burns calories even while you are resting. After all, your muscles are still using energy when you aren't actively working out.

If you build up your muscles, they will start to use energy faster, and you'll burn more calories without having to do anything to achieve this. Your resting metabolic rate will increase, and you should find it's a little easier to lose weight. It's important to be clear that this isn't going to make a phenomenal difference and you will still need to eat well and exercise regularly, but Pilates can improve how fast your body uses calories even when you're resting.

Pilates is therefore a great option for losing weight, especially if other forms of exercise are not open to you. For those who do undertake other forms of exercise, it can make an excellent complementary option, and will increase your ability in those other areas.

It's also fantastically good for your flexibility, balance, and posture, which is what we will look at next.

How pilates helps with
Flexibility, balance, and posture

Pilates is perhaps most famous for its ability to help with your flexibility, your balance, and your posture. This is one of the reasons that it is popular among elderly individuals, who may be struggling with these three areas, and suffering as a result.

It's important to be aware of how important of these three things are to your general well-being, so let's look at them in more detail. When these three areas are weak, you are at significantly higher risk of musculoskeletal injuries, which can be serious in some cases.

Flexibility

Loss of flexibility can impact your everyday activities, because it prevents you from bending, lifting, and moving with ease. Even activities like turning around, looking over your shoulder, or opening a cupboard can become challenging if your flexibility is particularly poor. This is true for individuals of all ages.

There's a greater risk of injuring yourself if you are not a flexible individual, too. This is because you may end up pulling joints or tearing muscles when you try to move. If your joints and muscles don't stretch very far before they get damaged, they are much more likely to get hurt when you're working out – or even just in day to day life.

Some people mistakenly think that you have to be naturally flexible in order to do Pilates, but this is definitely not the case. Pilates is designed to increase your flexibility. People who are naturally flexible may find it easier to complete some of the exercises, but if you persevere, you can increase your flexibility simply through consistent exercise. If you've always felt flexibility is something you're lacking, doing some Pilates could be the answer.

BALANCE

Balance is another key aspect of life, and having good balance reduces your risk of injuries and makes you more capable of undertaking activities. Balance is something that many people struggle with, but it's hard to overstate just how important this is to everyday tasks. Having a poor sense of balance can leave you at greater risk of falls and injuries.

Pilates is an excellent way to improve your balance, for a few different reasons. The most important is that it hones your core muscles, which gives you better poise and stability. You'll often be working out the muscles that you use when you are standing, which strengthens these muscles and makes it easier for you to find your centre of balance.

Pilates also works out muscles that you don't use everyday, but which benefit and support the muscles you do use. You might be astounded by how weak these stabilising muscles can be – and this is true for everyone, even individuals who exercise regularly and have good strength in their other muscles.

Boosting your stabiliser muscles again gives you improved balance and a better ability to stay upright, in a comfortable position, for longer. One of the great things about Pilates is that it offers a full body workout, so you'll be enhancing your abdominal strength, your leg strength, your arm strength, your chest strength, and more. This overall workout helps you to balance better.

Whatever age you are, good balance is key to protecting yourself from injuries, and it's something that can be challenging to attain. Committing to regular Pilates workouts is an excellent way to improve your overall balance by increasing your core strength, and the strength of your supporting muscles.

POSTURE

Good posture is also a very important part of your daily life. If your posture is poor, you'll end up suffering from a wide range of issues, including things like an aching back, stiff shoulders, a sore neck, etc.

These can lead to other problems, including difficulty standing up straight, limited arm mobility, headaches, and more. Having good posture is key to tackling and minimising these problems, but it is something that many people struggle to achieve.

Fortunately, if you have a strong core, you are more likely to enjoy good posture, because your body will naturally support itself in a better position. If the muscles in your back and stomach are weak, you will tend to hunch over, curling in on yourself, which can lead to habitually poor posture, and lots of problems.

Committing to doing Pilates regularly will help to address these issues, making you more comfortable and helping you to adopt a more upright stance in your everyday life.

As you can see, Pilates is a great exercise to adopt if you have any issues with your flexibility, balance, or posture – and we can all improve in these areas, even if they are already good! Wall Pilates may improve your quality of life and reduce your risk of injuries, so don't underestimate how valuable this form of exercise can be.

Next, we're going to spend a bit of time understanding why wall Pilates is such an effective form of exercise.

THE SCIENCE BEHIND WALL PILATES AND WHY IT IS SO EFFECTIVE

We all know that exercise in general is healthy, but why is Pilates a particularly good option? What makes this something you should consider including as part of your daily life? Let's find out more about this style of exercise.

Pilates is a mind-body exercise, meaning that it's thought to be beneficial to both your physical fitness and your mental health. The breathing component, which involves using your breath to increase your ability to stretch and move, is good for your mental health, and helps you to be fully absorbed in the exercise while undertaking it.

This form of exercise is focused almost exclusively on building your muscle strength and increasing your endurance. It's not about working out your cardiovascular system (which is why it is often paired with other forms of exercise to make it a well-rounded option).

Many Pilates techniques involve using your own body, or the wall, as a form of resistance. This minimises the risk of injury, and also makes this form of exercise more accessible, because you don't need any fancy equipment, a huge space, or to attend a class. You can do it from home, with just a wall and enough space to move around comfortably.

Pilates only started to gain real attention around the 1990s, and yet countless people have had their lives transformed by this style of exercise. It's also worth noting that surprisingly few studies have been done in this area, so there's a lot of scope for science to look into and better understand why Pilates tends to be effective.

Preliminary studies have suggested so far that it can:

- REDUCE CHRONIC PAIN
- IMPROVE FLEXIBILITY
- REDUCE ANXIETY AND DEPRESSION

- IMPROVE MUSCLE ENDURANCE
- INCREASE YOUR BALANCE

More work is needed to understand each of these areas, but let's explore them individually in more detail. Note that these studies looked at Pilates in general, rather than specifically wall Pilates, but we can still infer a significant amount from their findings.

REDUCING CHRONIC PAIN

A review of the literature surrounding Pilates was done in 2018, and it indicated that 19 out of 23 studies (from 2005 to 2016) had found Pilates more effective than control groups when it came to tackling various kinds of chronic pain.

The majority of trials done in recent years found that Pilates was an effective tool for rehabilitation, and was good at achieving the desired outcomes when dealing with physical disabilities and pain.

IMPROVING MUSCLE ENDURANCE

A study completed in 2010 (2) explored the ability of Pilates to increase muscular endurance, and it found that undertaking 60 minutes of Pilates twice per week for 12 weeks resulted in a significant increase of abdominal endurance.

Byrnes K, Wu PJ, Whillier S. Is Pilates an effective rehabilitation tool? A systematic review. J Bodyw Mov Ther. 2018 Jan;22(1):192-202. doi: 10.1016/j.jbmt.2017.04.008. Epub 2017 Apr 26. PMID: 2332746.

(2) Kloubec, June A. Pilates for Improvement of Muscle Endurance, Flexibility, Balance, and Posture. Journal of Strength and Conditioning Research 24(3):p 661-667, March 2010. | DOI: 10.1519/JSC.0b013e3181c277a6

IMPROVING FLEXIBILITY

The same study referenced above also looked into the effect of Pilates on flexibility, and found that hamstring flexibility was significantly improved when compared with the control group. This suggests that the exercise style can be used to increase flexibility in other areas too.

INCREASING YOUR BALANCE

We have already talked about how Pilates can boost your balance, and you can see evidence for this in Barker and Talevski's 2015 review. This review explored six studies that were aimed at testing whether Pilates exercises could reduce the risk of falls, and improve balance. On average, the participants were over 60 years old, and predominantly women.

Pilates was shown to improve balance in these adults, and one study also found that it was capable of reducing falls – although the other studies didn't look into this.

REDUCING ANXIETY AND DEPRESSION

Of course, it isn't all about physical fitness; some studies have suggested that doing Pilates can make you feel better mentally too. A 2018 analysis of existing studies suggested that while further research is needed, there is evidence to suggest that Pilates can improve your mental well-being and help you to feel better. It may be able to reduce stress, anxiety, and depression. (4)

----

(3) Barker, A.L., Bird, M. & Talevski, J. Effects of pilates exercise for improving balance in older adults: A systematic review with meta-analysis Archives of Physical Medicine and Rehabilitation. 2015;96:715-723

(4) K.M. Fleming, M.P. Herring, The effects of pilates on mental health outcomes: a meta-analysis of controlled trials, Complemen Therap Med, 37 (2018), pp. 80-95

This is true of exercise as a whole, but it tends to be particularly associated with exercises that involve the mind as well as the body, often using deep breathing techniques. Things like yoga, Tai chi, and Pilates are known for their ability to create a sense of calmness and tranquillity, and with this in mind, it's no wonder that Pilates is associated with reduced anxiety and depression.

It's certainly not a cure-all for everybody, but it's worth bearing in mind that there seem to be mental benefits as well as physical benefits when it comes to doing Pilates!

Before finishing this section, it's important to note that some of the studies done on Pilates so far have used relatively small control groups, and there's still a lot more to be done. Bear in mind that science hasn't necessarily caught up with the explosion of popularity that Pilates has enjoyed in recent years, and it is a surprisingly under-studied area, with only a handful of existing studies, many of which used small groups to research their findings.

We're still coming to understand this exercise style – but so far, all the evidence suggests that it's beneficial in many different ways! Next, let's look at how having a 21-day action plan can help you maximise the benefits you enjoy from Pilates.

THE BENEFITS OF FOLLOWING A 21-DAY PILATES ACTION PLAN AND WHAT TO EXPECT

When you first start a new kind of exercise, it's pretty easy to stay motivated and to do it every day or every two days. However, as the exercise gets "old" and your motivation drops, there's a risk that you will give up on the exercise, and either move on to something different, or stop exercising entirely. This is obviously something you'll want to avoid, and there's where the 21-day exercise plan comes in.

It's also important from another angle; it's easy to over-train when you have your initial burst of enthusiasm, and this can lead to injuries, especially if you aren't currently in great shape. Being injured will inevitably hamper your ability to stick with your exercise goals, and overall makes you less likely to continue exercising.

A 21-day action plan solves both of these issues by creating a paced, regular workout routine for you to stick to. By the time you've done 21 days of exercise, you're likely to have started building a habit, and this means you have a better chance of keeping up your Pilates routine. You'll also have built up your strength and learned to pace yourself, meaning that you're at less risk of overtraining.

Estimates on how long it takes to form a habit vary – and of course, different people need different periods. For some, 21 days will be enough, according to certain studies. That means you'll have made wall Pilates a regular part of your life, and you're more likely to continue doing it in the long term.

For others, it takes longer, and you might need approximately 60 to 70 days to form a habit. That can feel like a big commitment to begin with, though, and might seem overwhelming. It's therefore best to create a 21-day action plan, because this will form the building blocks of your exercise routine and make it easier for you to succeed.

When you reach the end of the 21 days, you can then increase the difficulty if you choose to, or simply repeat the routine until you feel like Pilates is a regular part of your life. Having the structure of a three-week cycle is a great way to help yourself "stick with it" in the long term.

For others, it takes longer, and you might need approximately 60 to 70 days to form a habit. That can feel like a big commitment to begin with, though, and might seem overwhelming. It's therefore best to create a 21-day action plan, because this will form the building blocks of your exercise routine and make it easier for you to succeed.

When you reach the end of the 21 days, you can then increase the difficulty if you choose to, or simply repeat the routine until you feel like Pilates is a regular part of your life. Having the structure of a three-week cycle is a great way to help yourself "stick with it" in the long term.

It's worth noting that many people find it particularly difficult to maintain their commitment to exercising around the 1 and 2 month marks, so you shouldn't just depend upon your 21-day plan for helping you meet your exercise goals. If you experience a dip at any point, feel free to change things up to increase your motivation, or spend some time reviewing your goals and your achievements so far, so you feel more inspired to continue.

Remember too that it's okay to take a workout break (not a rest day, but a deliberate break that lasts for at least several days) if you need one. This is when you choose to take time away from your normal exercise routine to deal with other priorities, let your body heal, or simply avoid burning out.

There are many 21-day plans online that you can follow if you choose to, or you can build your own if you would prefer. Simply use the exercises you find in this book to create a routine for yourself, and then put this somewhere visible, increasing the chances that you will follow it.

If you are going to create your own 21-day wall Pilates plan, there are a few things you should consider, including:

- Where you currently are in terms of your physical fitness, and what you are capable of initially

- Where you would like to be, how far this is from your current position, and how you can begin working in that direction

- What's realistic to achieve in the given timespan, and how you can ensure that you will achieve that

It's important to make sure that your exercise plan starts out easy, and has a difficulty curve. You don't want to challenge yourself too much at the start, but you do want to make sure that you are increasing the difficulty as your capacities grow. This will maximise the benefits you get from your exercise plan, and should ensure you don't get bored or start to stagnate.

To create a plan, you may find it helps to get a diary or simply to write out the next 21 days on a sheet of paper. For each day, make a note of what you plan to do on that day, and make sure you are varying your exercises to work out different muscles and give your body the appropriate rest. If you focus on your arms one day, focus on your legs or your abdomen the next.

Once you have created an exercise plan that you think will suit you, make sure you follow it, but don't be afraid to adjust it if you need to at times. It's okay to decide that you need to do more or less of certain exercises; you aren't creating a rigid set of rules that you must adhere to at all times. You're creating a plan to build your fitness, and it's good to adapt this if you need to.

You might be wondering what you can expect if you follow this kind of plan, and the answer is: consistent results. You'll start to see your body changing after a couple of weeks, and you should feel it too, as you adapt to the exercises and your muscles, flexibility, and balance improve. Consistency is the key, and this sort of plan will give you consistency.

Basic alignment and
Breathing techniques

Breathing and alignment are the absolute foundations of Pilates, and if you don't take the time to learn these properly, there's a high risk that you will never get the true benefit of this exercise style. You need to be able to breathe with your movements in order to stretch deeply, and you need your body to be in alignment so you don't hurt yourself.

It's therefore important to spend some time working on these things before you even begin your first Pilates exercise, and that's what we'll cover in this section. Feel free to come back and practise these techniques as often as you like; this will help you to feel more comfortable as you exercise.

Don't worry if you don't pick these up immediately. It can take some time and practise to get the hang of alignment and breathing, but you will gradually start to develop a sense of both of these, and you'll find your Pilates exercises far more enjoyable as a result. With that in mind, let's start with some basic alignment techniques.

Alignment

The alignment principle is about the way in which your major body parts (usually your ankles, your knees, your hips, your spine, your shoulders, and your head) relate to each other.

Take a few moments to think about how each of these body parts are currently related, as you sit reading this. Is your head at a strange angle with your shoulders? How straight is your spine? Are your hips and knees in line with each other, or skewed?

Of course, most of us don't naturally rest with all of our joints in line all of the time. However, your posture has a massive impact on the wear and tear that your muscles and joints endure, and thinking about it can make a significant difference to how you stand, sit, and move in everyday life, as well as during periods of exercise.

You can improve your alignment by making a point of thinking about this regularly. Consider the way that you move, and how all these body parts relate to each other as you do so. Try to pull those parts back into line when you notice that they are slipping out.

For example, if you realise you frequently stand with your head tipped to the side, you're probably putting strain on the muscles in your neck, and this may eventually result in an injury. You might be clenching your teeth when stressed, which is putting strain on your neck muscles, and having a knock-on effect on your spine. Tension can run a surprisingly long way through your body, and constant tension will result in stress, soreness, and muscle damage.

You can reduce this risk by consciously checking how you are standing or moving whenever you undertake an activity, and making an effort to pull your joints back into line with each other. Sometimes, just being aware of your basic alignment is sufficient for helping you improve it.

However, if you're not finding that enough, try imagining that you are a puppet, and all your joints are connected to each other by strings. For example, your knees are connected to your hips by strings. You want those strings to be straight, not tangled, and reasonably relaxed, rather than taut.

Practising alignment can be very challenging at first, but it's important to keeping working on it and thinking about it. Gradually, you will find that your alignment improves, and it becomes second nature to balance your joints and hold your body in a way that minimises stress. This will also make exercises easier and more beneficial, reducing the amount of stress that they put on your body.

Alignment is one of the core principles of Pilates, so don't underestimate its importance, and don't dismiss it as a waste of time.

In this book, we're going to talk about getting into alignment in most of the exercises. What alignment means will vary from exercise to exercise, but the overall principle remains the same: think about how your joints relate to each other, and draw straight lines in between them.

For example, if you extend a foot out in front of you, your foot will generally remain in line with your knee, which will remain in line with your hip. Similarly, if you extend an arm, your hand will remain aligned with your elbow, which will remain aligned with your shoulder. Thinking about how all your joints relate to each other as you move around will increase your alignment, and the overall benefit that you get from the exercise.

A basic aligned position will involve standing upright with your feet, knees, hips, and shoulders all in line with each other, and your arms by your sides. You'll see variations of this position throughout the book, and many exercises start from this point.

BREATHING TECHNIQUES

Breathing is as important as alignment in Pilates, and Joseph Pilates himself emphasised how critical this is to every aspect of Pilates exercises. It is possibly the most fundamental principle.

If you are not familiar with breathing exercises, it's a good time to spend some time simply sitting and practising some techniques before you begin exercising. It can take some time to get used to thinking about and controlling your breathing, and it's harder to do this if you are also focusing on moving your body in new ways. Instead of trying to combine breathing and exercise initially, make a commitment to practising some breathing exercises for 5-10 minutes every day, until this becomes easier and more natural for you.

You can practise at any time of day, whatever you are doing. Try this while you're washing up, cleaning your home, sitting at your desk, going for a walk, or reading a book. It can take a surprising amount of focus, but once you've mastered some techniques, you'll find that it comes much more easily.

If you already do other breathing-related exercises (such as yoga), you may find that this is pretty straightforward, but it's still a good idea to do some practise. To fully unlock the benefits of Pilates, you need to be able to breathe effectively.

Pilates involves the following technique:

• Breathing in through the nose, and expanding the ribs laterally

• Breathing out through the mouth, and drawing the ribs in and down.

You should find that your ribcage moves and expands when you breathe in, rather than your abdomen expanding. This will help to keep your abdominal muscles activated while you're exercising, while breathing into the abdomen makes it harder to ensure they are active. You cannot easily contract your abdominal muscles if they are expanding and contracting with your breath.

You also want to make sure that your ribs don't flare forwards when you breathe in, because this will make it much harder to keep your oblique muscles active. These stabilise your spine, so keeping them active is important for safety while you are doing Pilates.

Instead, your ribs should expand laterally, and when you breathe out, your ribs should move down towards your hips, keeping the obliques active.

If you are struggling with this technique, try watching some videos online to see exactly how another person undertakes it. It's worth taking the time to properly learn how to breathe, because you'll make your Pilates exercises more rewarding and enjoyable, and they'll be safer too.

Once you've mastered basic alignment and a good breathing technique, it's time to start exercising – so in the next section, we'll cover the warm-ups you can do.

WARM-UP EXERCISES:
PREPARE YOUR BODY AND MIND FOR SUCCESS

Warming up is a key part of any exercise routine, and Pilates is no exception. You might think that because it's a relatively gentle form of exercise (compared with some other options), you don't need to warm up, but that's absolutely not the case. Warming up is critically important.

You're going to be asking your muscles to move and stretch in unusual ways, and you need to make sure that they are warm enough to stretch effectively, or you risk tears and strains. The better you warm up before you begin your exercise routine, the less likely you are to hurt yourself, and the less stiffness you will experience after the exercise.

A warm-up can be quick and easy, but it is crucial. Try some of these exercises.

WARM-UP 1
SIDE STRETCHES

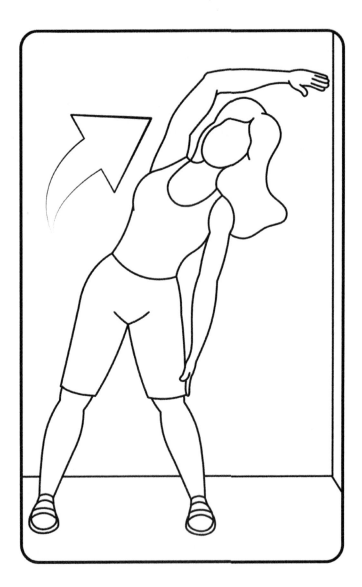

1.) Get into a comfortable, aligned position, with your hands by your sides.

2.) Gradually lift your right arm up out to the side, holding it out straight. Lift it further, until it arches over your head, and begin to bend with it, so that your body curves towards the wall. Avoid leaning forwards or backwards; you are just trying to curve to the side.

3.) As you move your right arm upwards and arc your body, gently slide your left arm down, against your leg.

4.) Keep arching sideways until you feel the stretch in the right-hand side of your body. You may be able to touch your right hand to the wall on your left, or this may be too much of a stretch – just go as far as feels comfortable to you.

5.) When you have reached the point where the stretch feels good, stay there for a few seconds, and then arch your arm back and return to the aligned position with your hands by your sides.

6.) Repeat this motion 5 times.

7.) Next, turn around so your right shoulder faces the wall, and repeat the stretch with your left arm arching over your head, and the left side of your body stretching over to the right.

8.) Repeat this 5 times to finish the stretch.

Warm-up 2
Leg Lifts

1.) Stand with your back against a wall in a neutral position, with your legs the same distance apart as your hips. Put your hands on your hips.

2.) Lift your right leg up into the air, and form a right angle with your calves and quads.

3.) Lift until your quads are parallel with the floor if you can, keeping your calves at a right angle. Hold this position for a few seconds.

4.) Return your foot to the floor, and then repeat the exercise with your left leg.

5.) Do this 5 times with each leg.

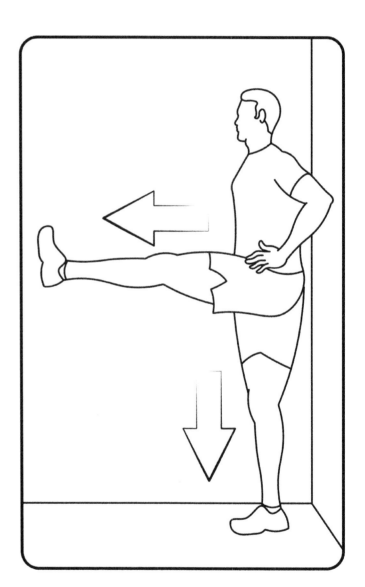

Warm-up 3
Pulses

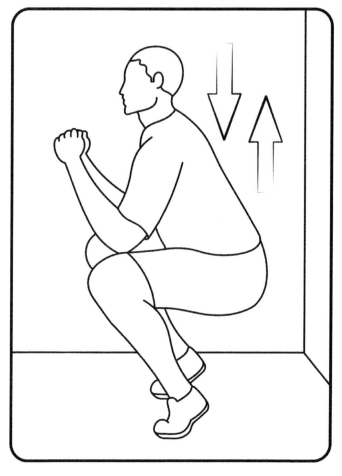

1.) Stand with your back against the wall for support, assuming a neutral position with all your joints in line.

2.) Place your hands on your hips, and then lower into a slight squat. You may need to take half a step away from the wall to do this comfortably, but make sure you remain upright as you dip into the squat.

3.) Lift back up, and then dip down again. Repeat this up to 10 times, engaging the muscles at the tops of your thighs and hips.

4.) Return to a neutral position.

WARM-UP 4
NECK STRETCH

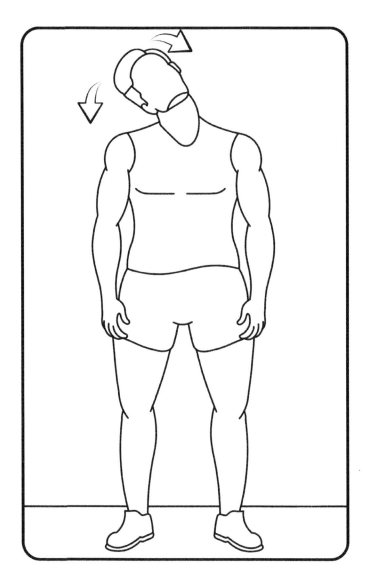

1.) Stand with your back to a wall, and your hands at your sides. Make sure your joints are aligned.

2.) Touch the back of your head against the wall, and then begin to gently tilt it down to the left, still looking forwards. The goal is for your left ear to touch your left shoulder, but you must avoid hunching your shoulder up towards your head to achieve this. Keep your shoulder level, and only go as far as feels comfortable to you.

3.) Lift your head back into the neutral position, and then lower it down towards your left shoulder again. Repeat this 5 times, and then swap to the same exercise for the right-hand side.

4.) When you have completed 5 stretches on the right, gently roll your neck so that your chin drops towards your chest and then comes up on the left, and then roll it back to the right.

5.) Return to the central position and relax.

WARM-UP 5
SPINAL ROLL

1.) Stand with your back against a wall in a neutral position, with your legs the same distance apart as your hips. Put your hands on your hips.

2.) Lift your right leg up into the air, and form a right angle with your calves and quads.

3.) Lift until your quads are parallel with the floor if you can, keeping your calves at a right angle. Hold this position for a few seconds.

4.) Return your foot to the floor, and then repeat the exercise with your left leg.

5.) Do this 5 times with each leg.

4.) Return your foot to the floor, and then repeat the exercise with your left leg.

5.) Do this 5 times with each leg.

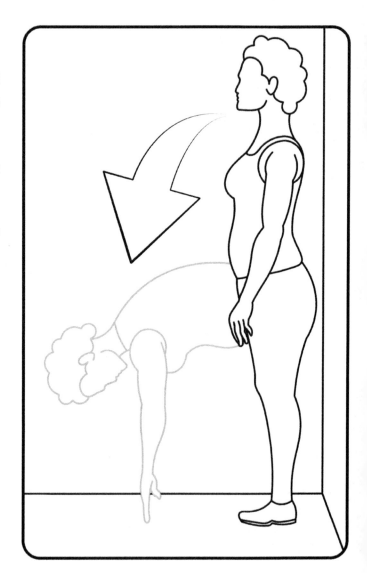

BEGINNER WALL
PILATES EXERCISES

In this section, we'll cover some of the simpler wall Pilates exercises that you might wish to try out. There are some great options here, and they are all ones that you should be able to at least attempt even at the beginning of your fitness journey.

Note that if you do find something too challenging, it's better not to push too hard. Have a go at it, and then move on to a different exercise and return to the difficult one another day. Gradually building up your skills, confidence, strength, and flexibility is essential to ensuring that you don't hurt yourself when it comes to wall Pilates, especially if you are a beginner.

With that in mind, let's get started!

Exercise 1
Standing Lunge

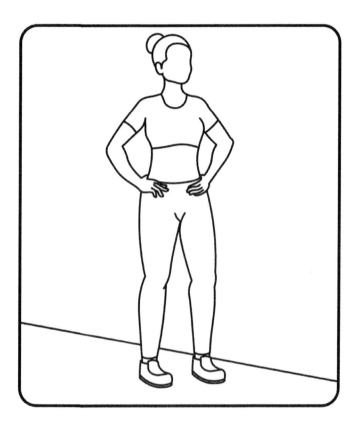

3.) Straighten your upper body and lift your chest so that your legs are taking the stretch, rather than any other part of your body. Find your centre of balance. If you feel comfortable, you can lift your hand off the wall, but you don't need to.

4.) Slowly straighten your left leg by lifting with the muscles just beneath your buttock. Avoid lifting with your knee, as this may injure it.

5.) Hold the position for 30 seconds, making sure your joints are in line, your pelvis is square, and you feel comfortable and balanced.

6.) Lift back into the central position, and then swap legs so you are stretching your other hip.

1.) Position yourself so that you are standing tall, with your right shoulder facing the nearest wall. This wall is going to provide you with support, so place your right hand on it. Check all of your joints are in line.

2.) Bend your right knee, and step back with your left foot. Make sure your pelvis remains square, and doesn't twist as you move. Keep your right hand on the wall, and rest your left hand on your hip or thigh, but don't press down. Gently sink down to stretch your legs.

EXERCISE 2
TURNOUT SQUATS

1.) Stand with your left shoulder facing towards the wall, and place one hand on the wall. Get your body into alignment.

2.) Put your feet in a Pilates V. Your heels should be touching, while your toes turn out from your body, forming a V shape. Find a comfortable centre of balance in this position.

3.) Inhale as you bend your knees, keeping your back straight to come into a squat. Make sure you keep your heels together, and avoid moving your feet. Keep your hand on the wall.

4.) Exhale to come back up, and then inhale to squat again.

5.) Keep repeating this about 10 times, working out the muscles in your calves. If you find it's uncomfortable initially, repeat it just 5 times, and scale up gradually.

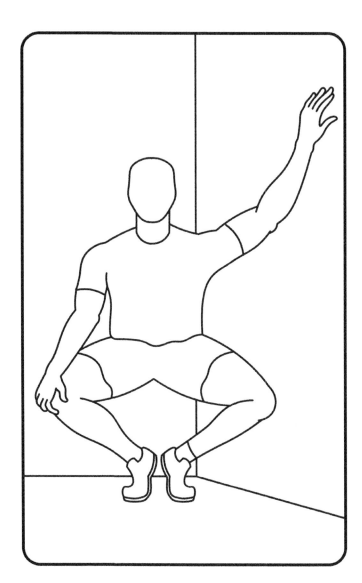

Exercise 3
Standing Crunches

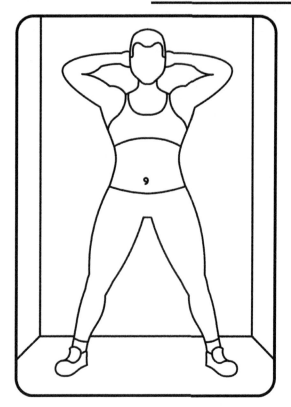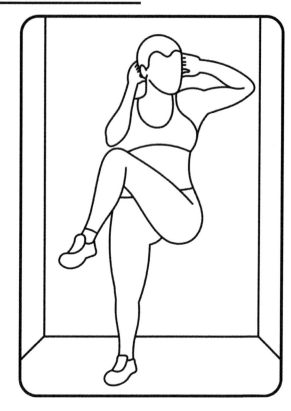

1.) Stand up in an aligned position, and place your hands behind your head, with your elbows bent. Again, you may find that it helps to have a wall against your back for support.

2.) Press your elbows outwards behind you so that they come close to the wall, and gradually lift your right leg up towards your torso. Your knee should face outwards.

3.) Slowly bend towards your knee, so that your core muscles stretch. Find the deepest stretch that is comfortable for you, hold it for a few seconds, and then return your leg to the floor and straighten up until your elbows touch the wall again.

4.) Repeat this with your left leg, and complete the exercise 3 times on each side.

INTERMEDIATE WALL
PILATES EXERCISES

If you're ready to take it up a notch, here are some slightly more challenging wall Pilates exercises that you might like to try.

Exercise 1
Footwork Parallel

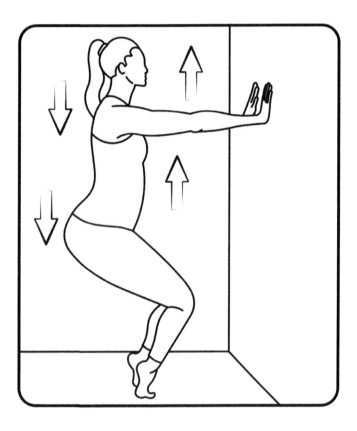

You will reach a position where it feels like you are about to sit in a chair. Pause here to check your alignment is good.

5.) Once you are comfortable, lift your heels slightly, keeping your pelvis level.

6.) Press into the balls of your feet and further lift your heels. You can now straighten your legs, sliding your hands back up the wall as your body lifts.

7.) Lower your heels back onto the floor, keeping your body nice and straight. Your body shouldn't move much; your calf muscles will stretch out to let your heels move.

8.) Repeat this exercise 3 times.

1.) Stand facing a wall, with your feet and legs parallel, and your knees soft.

2.) Place your palms on the wall so that you can support yourself.

3.) Engage your abdominal muscles, and gradually start to lengthen your spine. Reach the top of your head towards the ceiling, and pull your buttocks down towards the floor.

4.) Slide your hands down the wall as you move, bending your knees and keeping your shoulders relaxed.

EXERCISE 2
WALL HAMSTRING STRETCH

1.) Lie on your mat, with your bottom close to the wall, and your legs up the wall, the soles of your feet facing the ceiling. You can put a cushion under your bottom if this feels more comfortable. Find a neutral, aligned position, opening your chest.

2.) Once you are comfortable and ready to start, flex your feet, and keep your left leg and left side very still.

3.) Reach your arms out on either side of you and press them onto the mat. Push into your hands to give yourself stability.

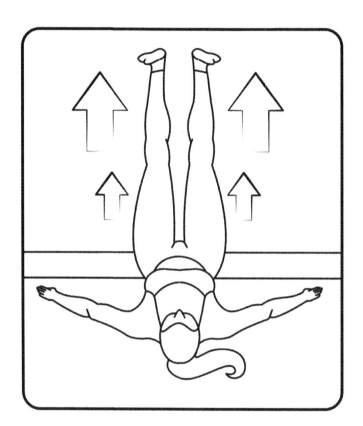

4.) Inhale and slowly begin to slide your right leg to the right, keeping the rest of your body as still as possible. Make sure this movement is controlled, and your bottom remains resting on the floor, so only your leg is moving.

5.) Go as far as feels comfortable, and then stop and hold the position for a couple of seconds.

6.) Exhale and pull the leg back to the central position, using your core muscles to pull the leg in.

7.) Repeat this, making sure that your left leg stays still and your bottom stays against the ground. You should do 5 repetitions on the right side, and then swap to the left side, and do 5 repetitions on that side.

Exercise 3
Shoulder Stretch

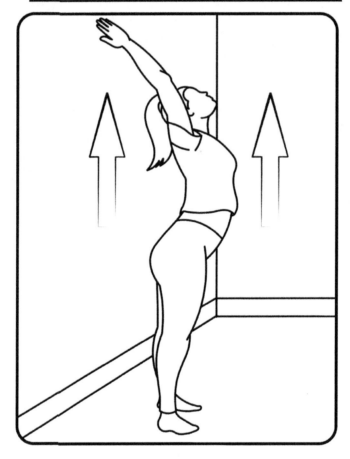

1.) Stand close to the wall, not touching it, with your back to it. Bring your body into alignment, and then reach your arms up in front of you.

2.) Bring them back over your head, so that your fingers brush the wall, and your elbows are a little higher than your head.

3.) Once you are comfortable in this position, take a small step away from the wall, but keep your hands on it to create a stretch. Arch your body into a C shape. Press against the wall with your hands to tension the muscles.

4.) Step back against the wall, bending your arms as you bring your body in again.

5.) Step away, and then back against the wall another 3 times, pressing into the wall throughout the exercise.

ADVANCED WALL
PILATES EXERCISES

Now, here are some of the more advanced options you might want to consider trying.

EXERCISE 1
WALL WALK DOWN INTO BRIDGE

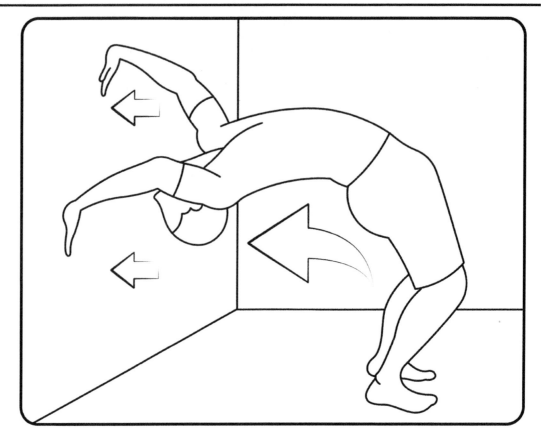

1.) As with the previous exercise, you will start by standing with your back to the wall, your hands at your sides.

2.) Raise your arms in front of you, and then lift them up, over your head, and touch the wall behind you.

3.) Step away from the wall, arching your body so you can keep your hands against the wall. Widen your legs to give yourself more balance if necessary.

4.) Start walking your hands down the wall, bending your back. Go slowly and give yourself time to adjust. You may need to shuffle your feet to maintain this position.

5.) When you reach the floor, you will be in the bridge position. Hold this for a few seconds, and then gradually walk your hands back up the wall until you are standing upright again.

6.) Repeat this 3 to 5 times.

EXERCISE 2
FEET ON THE WALL

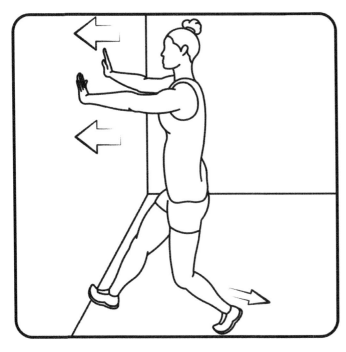

1.) Start by standing about a pace away from the wall. Lean back until your back is in contact with the wall, and your legs are angled in front of you, your feet flat on the floor.

2.) Inhale and sweep your arms out to the sides and then up over your head.

3.) Swing your arms downwards, following them with your head and upper body, until you are almost able to touch your feet, and only your bottom remains touching the wall.

4.) If necessary, adjust your feet and find your centre of balance, and then remove your weight from the wall and shift so that you are standing on your feet, with your fingertips touching the floor.

5.) Soften your knees so that you can place your hands flat on the floor comfortably. Bend the knees and straighten them a few times to exercise the hip muscles.

6.) Next, with your knees slightly bent, lift your left leg off the floor and up behind you. Place your foot against the wall as high up as feels comfortable. If you cannot touch the wall, feel free to move a little further away, until you find a comfortable position.

7.) Straighten your left leg against the wall, and simultaneously try to straighten your right leg (the one your weight is on) a little bit.

8.) Hold this for 3 seconds, and then bring your leg back down and beneath your body. Bend your knees.

9.) Swap to the other leg, lifting it up as high against the wall as feels comfortable, and then straightening your legs. Hold for 3 seconds, and return to the central position.

10.) Do this 4 times on each side.

Exercise 3
Full Feet On The Wall Inversion

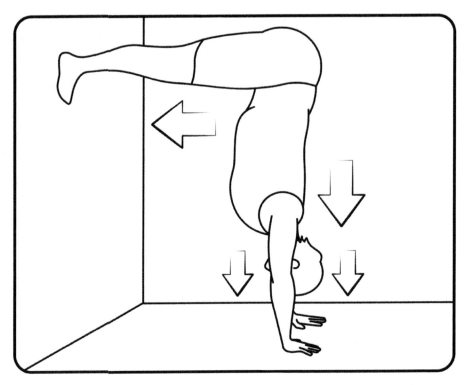

1.) Start about a pace and a half away from the wall, facing away from it. Stand in a neutral, aligned position. Put your feet together, with about an inch between them.

2.) Sweep your arms around and place your palms on the floor, bending your knees if you need to. Your hands should be directly under your shoulders, with your feet just behind them, still almost touching.

3.) Lift your left leg up and walk it onto the wall behind you, as high as feels comfortable to you. Get your foot against the wall so you can support yourself and balance. Shift your hands until you feel comfortable and safe.

4.) Next, lift the right leg, and place your right foot on the wall beside your left foot. Again, shift until you feel comfortable and you have found your balance.

5.) Walk both feet slowly down until your body reaches a 90 degree angle, with your body parallel with the wall.

6.) Hold this position for a few seconds, and then lower your left leg to the floor and let your right leg come down too. Repeat a couple of times.

WALL PILATES EXERCISES FOR WEIGHT LOSS

For some people, losing weight is the ultimate goal, and there are some great exercises out there for this, too. Let's explore a few.

EXERCISE 1
WALL LIFTS

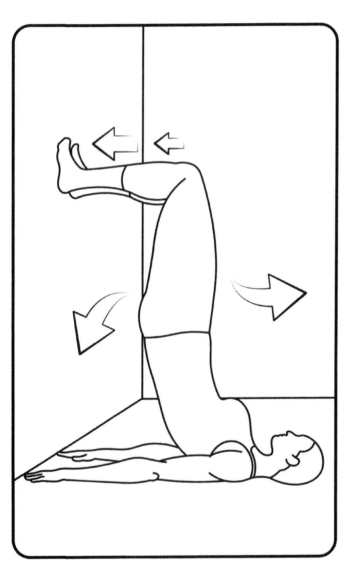

1.) Lie down on a mat with your feet facing towards the wall, and your body supine. Your palms should be facing the mat so you can use your arms if necessary.

2.) Slide yourself close to the wall, and place your feet on it, at around hip height (if you were standing). Both soles should be flat against the wall. Your knees should be level with your feet and form a right angle with your hips.

3.) From there, use your core muscles to lift your lower body up off the mat, pushing your feet into the wall. Hold for 3 seconds, and then lower back to the mat.

4.) Repeat this approximately 10 times.

Exercise 2
Wall Push-Ups

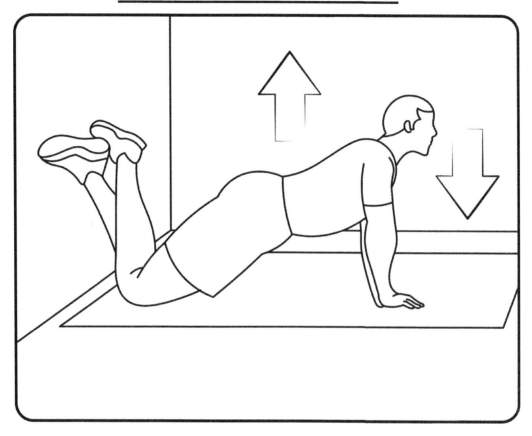

1.) Lie on your stomach on the mat, with your knees against the bottom of the wall and your calves and feet parallel to the wall.

2.) Put your palms approximately level with your ribcage, and use the muscles of your arms to lift your torso off the mat, in a modified push-up. Lift as much of your body as you feel comfortable with, but make sure your feet and calves remain against the wall, and don't slip out of alignment with your knees and hips.

3.) Repeat this 5 to 10 times.

EXERCISE 3
WALKING BRIDGE

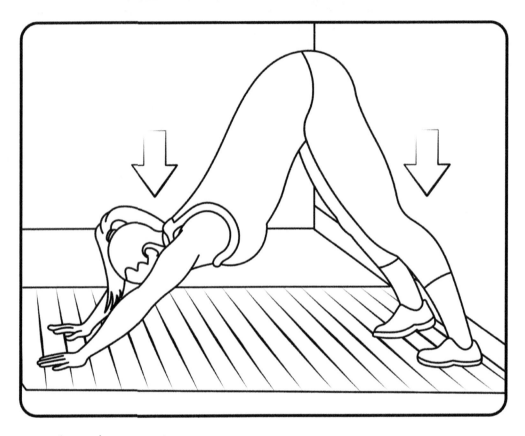

1.) Again, lie on your stomach on a mat.

2.) Start with your feet against the wall, and your hands on the mat in front of you. All of your joints should be in line, and your body should be approximately parallel with the floor, your head a little higher than your feet.

3.) Gradually walk your hands back towards your feet, arching your body up into an inverted V as you move. Go as far as feels comfortable for you, and hold for 3 seconds.

4.) Walk your hands back out away from your feet, letting your body follow to return to a plank-like position.

5.) Repeat this up to 10 times.

EXERCISE 4
SEATED ARM STRETCHES

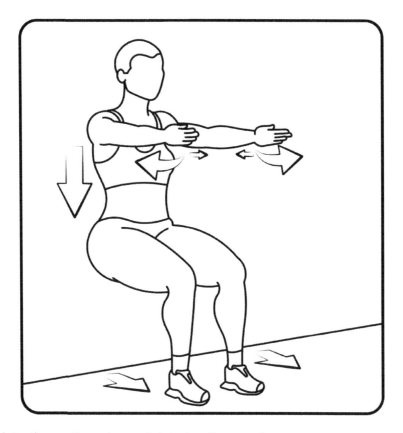

1.) Stand with your back to the wall, and your joints in alignment.

2.) Walk your feet forward while sliding your back down the wall, keeping contact with the wall. You are aiming for a seated position, where you are essentially sitting in mid-air, with the wall serving as your support. Your legs will be bent, with your feet a short distance behind your knees.

3.) Once you reach this position, you are going to hold it. Lift your arms up on either side of your body, and then bring them forward in front of you so that your palms touch. Keep the rest of your body as still as possible.

4.) Sweep your arms back out to the sides, and then bring them back to the centre.

5.) Repeat this for as long as you feel comfortable holding the position, and then gradually straighten up.

WALL PILATES EXERCISES FOR FLEXIBILITY

Improving your flexibility can revolutionise how comfortable you feel in everyday life. Lots of Pilates exercises will do this, but here are a few that are particularly effective.

EXERCISE 1
SIDE BEND

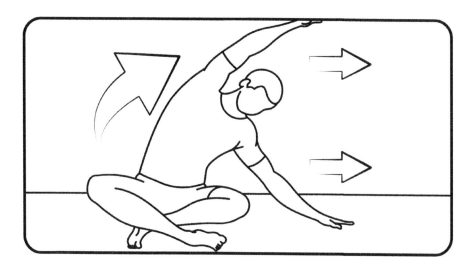

1.) Sit on the floor cross-legged, with your back against the wall, and get comfortable with your spine in a neutral position. If it helps, you can sit on a cushion to elevate your back and give your spine an opportunity to straighten out a little. The back of your head should touch the wall, or a cushion if you find touching the wall is uncomfortable.

2.) Next, walk your right hand out to the right, until it is slightly extended but your fingertips are still touching the floor.

3.) Bring your left arm straight up, with your palm facing inwards, towards your right-hand side. Lift up through your spine, until you are sitting as tall as you can. Lift the crown of your head, but keep your chin level.

4.) Pull your ribcage back towards the wall, and then begin to slide to your right. Walk your right hand outwards away from your body, while your left hand arcs with your body to provide a side stretch. Keep your hips still, so your side muscles are doing the work, rather than your hip muscles.

5.) Lengthen your body as much as possible, so you aren't crunching over on your right-hand abdominal muscles. Your goal is to pull your left hand up above your head on the right-hand side, rather than reaching it towards the mat on the right-hand side.

6.) Draw a deep breath in, and then roll your body back to the upright position. Repeat this twice on this side, and then swap sides so you are stretching your left instead.

EXERCISE 2
LEGS UP THE WALL

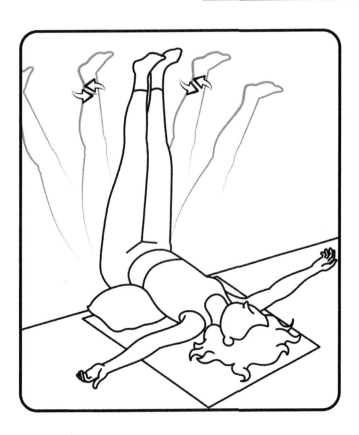

1.) Sit with your left shoulder facing the wall and your knees bent in front of you.

2.) Roll sideways onto your back, so that your feet end up against the wall, with a small gap between your bottom and the base of the wall. The soles of your feet should face the ceiling, a little closer together than the width of your hips.

3.) Rotate your legs gently back and forth, moving the whole leg (thighs, calves, and feet). You will see your feet turn away from each other and then back towards each other, along with the rest of the leg.

4.) Move your feet to just past shoulder-width apart, and bend your knees a little.

5.) Repeat the rotating movements, turning your joints towards and away from each other. Try to keep your pelvis still, so your hips, knees, and feet are the only parts of your body that are moving. This works out the hip joints more thoroughly.

6.) Straighten your knees gently (they can still be soft, but should no longer be bent) and take your legs slightly further apart, continuing the internal and external rotating movements. Stay here for a few rotations.

7.) Bring your legs a little further apart still, continuing to rotate them inwards and outwards, and remembering to keep your feet flexed so your toes are pointing towards the floor.

8.) Do this until you hit your comfort point, working in gradual increments to give your hips time to open up.

9.) When you hit the final point, gradually start bringing your legs back in to the central point, pausing to rotate every few increments.

EXERCISE 3
CAT STRETCHING

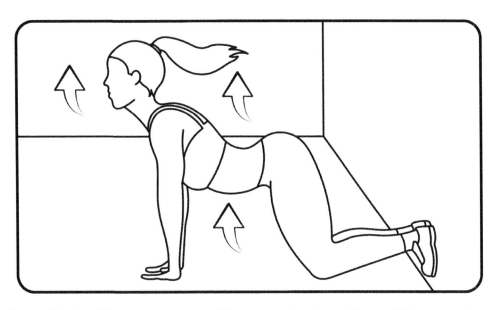

1.) Stand facing the wall, about two paces away. Place your hands on the wall for support.

2.) Line all of your joints up, and then bend your knees so you are slightly crouching, with your back straight and angled towards the wall.

3.) Draw in a deep breath, and then exhale and round your spine into a curve. This involves arching your back outwards like a cat stretching, and tucking your chin and buttocks in. You will end up looking towards the floor.

4.) As you inhale, press against the wall and arch your back inwards, lifting your head up towards the ceiling. Your spine will curve in the opposite direction. Keep your knees slightly bent.

5.) Exhale and round your back again, lowering your head down so you are looking at the floor again.

6.) Repeat this 4-5 times.

WALL PILATES

EXERCISES FOR POSTURE

Again, a lot of Pilates exercises will improve your general posture, because they make you more aware of your body and its movements – but in this section, we'll check out a few of the best techniques for you to try.

EXERCISE 1
FLAMINGO

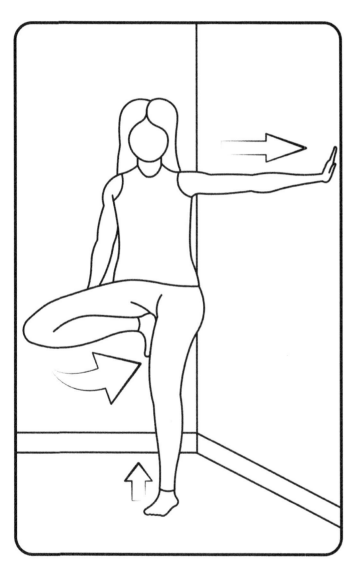

1.) Stand so your left shoulder is facing the wall, and place your left hand on the wall for balance.

2.) Lift your right leg off the floor, bend your knee, and place your foot against your left leg, as high up as feels comfortable to you. This may be against your calf, your knee, or even your upper thigh.

3.) Open up your hip so that you feel the stretch, and make sure your body is upright and tall. Hold for 10 seconds.

4.) Lower your foot back to the floor in a controlled motion, and repeat 2 more times.

5.) Swap legs and do the same exercise 3 times on the other side.

EXERCISE 2
WALL SITS

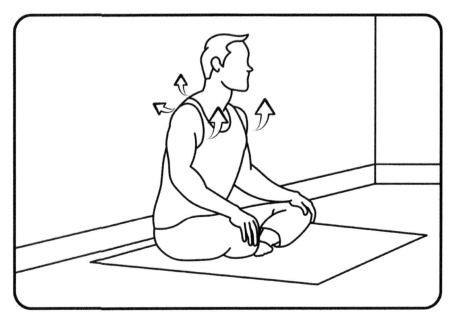

1.) Sit cross-legged on the floor with your back against the wall, aiming to get your back as straight as possible. If you find that your lower back is very rounded, place a light cushion underneath your bottom, and this should help you to straighten your spine. You can also place a pillow behind your head if you need to in order to straighten your neck.

2.) Sit in a neutral position, keeping your chin level. Open your chest up, and pull your ribcage back towards the wall.

3.) Lift your abdomen, and press your tailbone against the wall. Most of your posterior should now be touching the wall, except for a space between your neck and the wall, and your lower back and the wall.

4.) Gently lift your spine, without tilting your chin, to lengthen the vertebrae. You'll feel the stretch throughout your hip flexors and abs.

5.) Hold it for 10 seconds, and then relax a little, but do not slump.

6.) Reengage the muscles, lifting your spine without tilting your chin, and hold for another 10 seconds.

7.) Repeat this 5-10 times.

Exercise 3
Head & Shoulders Correction

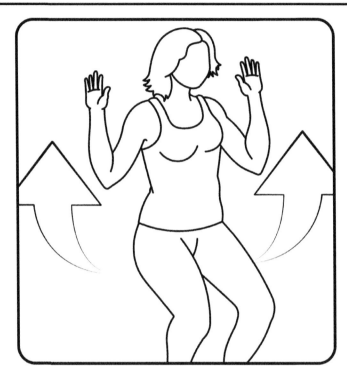

1.) Stand approximately one small step away from the wall, and then lean your body back so that your bottom touches the wall.

2.) Lean your back into the wall, straightening your spine gently, until you are resting most of your weight against the wall. Take a moment to think about how your shoulders are sitting, and whether they are rounding inwards.

3.) Breathe in, and then as you release the breath, draw your shoulders back and touch your palms to the wall. You can keep your arms by your sides, making sure that as much of them as possible touches the wall. Hold this position for approximately 3 breaths.

4.) Raise the arms up a little way, settling them about halfway between the shoulder and the hip on either side of your body, and then repeat the process of drawing your shoulders back and touching the wall. Hold the position for 3 breaths.

5.) Raise your palms up to shoulder height, turning them to face outwards. Keep your shoulders and arms against the wall, and complete another 3 breaths to stretch the front of your shoulders.

Wall Pilates
EXERCISES FOR BALANCE

A lot of the exercises we have already covered will improve your balance, but let's spend some time looking at a few that are specifically designed to help in this area.

Before you start doing these exercises, make sure you take the relevant safety precautions, especially if your balance isn't particularly good at the moment. As well as using the wall for support, you may also wish to have a sturdy chair that you can place a hand on if you need to. Work on a reasonably soft surface (such as a mat) so you are less likely to hurt yourself if you do fall.

Remember not to push yourself beyond your comfort zone when working on balance exercises. It's better to take a gradual approach and build up your skills than to risk falling and hurting yourself.

EXERCISE 1
ANKLE MOBILITY

1.) Stand facing the wall, and place your hands on it at around stomach or chest height. Get your feet approximately hip distance apart.

2.) Lift up onto your toes, using just the muscles in your ankles and lower legs, and not pressing with your arms.

3.) Lift up as high as feels comfortable, keeping your upper body straight. You can lightly lean on the wall if you need to for balance, but try to find a comfortable position where you aren't depending upon it too much.

4.) Drop gently back down onto your feet in a controlled fashion, and then raise up again.

5.) Repeat this exercise 6 to 7 times, breathing deeply. If you find yourself tipping to one side, use the wall to support yourself more, but focus on moving slowly and finding your balance independently.

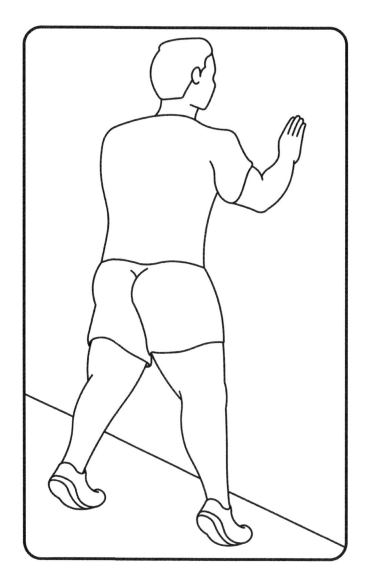

EXERCISE 2
WALKING IN PLACE

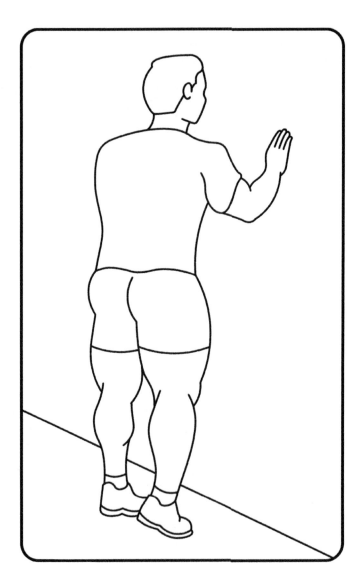

Note that this is an extension of the previous exercise, so you may wish to join the two together, or do them independently.

1.) Maintain your position, with your hands resting on the wall, and your body aligned.

2.) Come up onto your toes, keeping your hands on the wall.

3.) Bend your right knee, lowering your left heel to the ground at the same time. Get your foot completely flat on the floor, stretching the calf.

4.) Raise your left heel off the ground, bending the knee, and simultaneously lower your right heel to the ground, until it is flat on the floor.

5.) Keep swapping from side to side, almost as though you were walking on the spot. You should feel your head and upper body lift every time you swap from one foot to the other. Keep your upper body straight and upright.

6.) Do approximately 10 steps on each side.

Exercise 3
Leg Lifts

1.) Stand facing the wall, and place your palms on it, at about shoulder height. Get the rest of your body into alignment and find your centre of balance.

2.) Shift your weight onto your right leg.

3.) Lift your left foot off the floor and bring your left knee up towards the wall, forming a right angle. Hold it there for 10 seconds, and then lower it back to the floor.

4.) Swap so that your weight is on your left leg.

5.) Lift your right leg off the floor and bring your right knee up towards the wall, again forming a right angle. Hold it there for 10 seconds, and then lower it to the floor.

6.) Repeat on both sides 5 times.

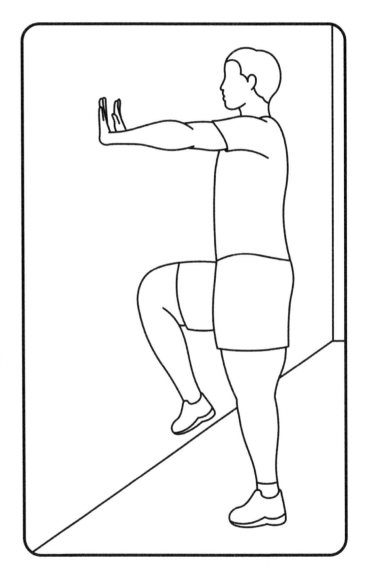

Exercise 4
Calf Stretch

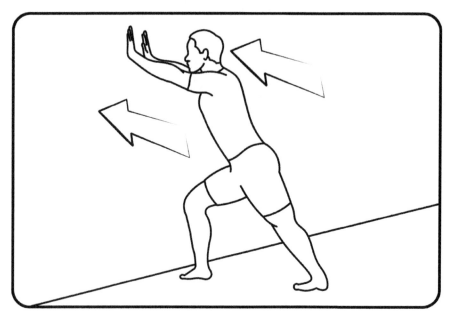

1.) Stand facing the wall, with your right foot half a step forward from your left foot, and the rest of your body in alignment. Rest your hands on the wall for support.

2.) Step your left foot back, bending your right knee and straightening your left leg so that your left heel touches the floor. This should create a gentle stretch.

3.) Shift your weight onto your right leg so that you can support yourself.

4.) Bring your left knee in towards the wall, so that it passes your right knee and almost touches the wall, and then stretch it back out behind you so that your toes touch the floor.

5.) Bring your left knee in again, and then stretch it out behind you again. You can move your body as you move your leg to increase your balance, but try not to let your other joints come out of alignment with each other; you should remain facing the wall squarely.

6.) Repeat this 5 times with your left knee, and then swap sides.

7.) Repeat the calf stretch with your right leg, heel touching the floor, and then put your weight on your left leg and bring your right knee in towards the wall. Stretch it back out behind you, and repeat this stretch 5 times.

PARTNER WALL PILATES EXERCISES

If you want to engage in Pilates exercises with a friend, you can also do this. It's a great way to give yourself more motivation, hold yourself accountable, and make exercising more fun — so let's look at how to approach this!

It's worth noting that in many cases, partners are used to replace the wall (providing the resistance and support that the wall might otherwise provide) so there aren't many of these exercises, but you can always adapt the other exercises in this book to create your own if you have some good ideas.

EXERCISE 1
TWISTS WITH A FRIEND

1.) Stand with your right shoulder facing a wall. Your partner needs to stand with their left shoulder facing the same wall, so you are looking at each other. The wall will provide guidance.

2.) Give your hands to your partner, and then draw in a deep breath and turn just your torso to the left. Your partner will hold onto your hands and provide resistance. Keep turning until you feel the stretch in your muscles.

3.) Turn back to face your partner, and then repeat the twist a further 3 times.

4.) Allow your partner to do the same number of turns while you hold their hands and provide the resistance. Check that they are not turning their hips, legs, or knees, and only their upper body is twisting.

5.) Swap places with your partner, and then rejoin hands and turn your torso to the right this time. Again, you should do this 3 or 4 times.

6.) Allow your partner to do their twists to the right.

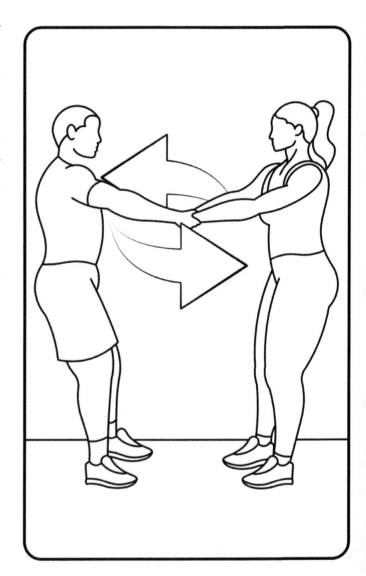

Exercise 2
Curls With A Friend

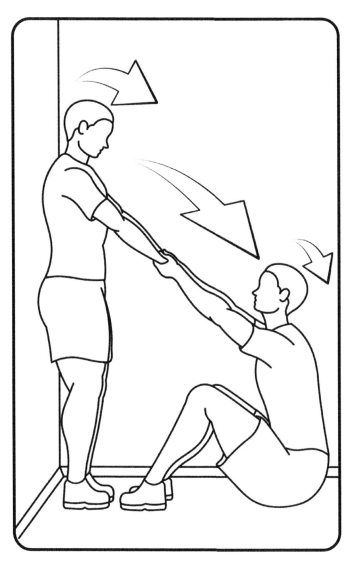

1.) Face your partner, with your back to the wall.

2.) Slide yourself close to the wall, and place your feetYour partner sits on the floor in front of you, with their knees bent, and their toes touching your toes.

3.) Join hands with your partner, and then inhale and begin to curl your body down towards the mat, starting from your chin.

4.) At the same time, your partner can lean backwards towards the floor, still holding your hands. Both of your bodies will provide resistance to each other. Go as far as feels comfortable for both of you.

5.) Once you have reached a limit, gradually start to straighten back up, while your partner sits up. Continue providing gentle resistance on both sides to test your muscles. You should reach the upright position at around the same time as your partner reaches the sitting position.

6.) You can repeat this a couple of times, and then swap places.

EXERCISE 3
DIPS WITH A FRIEND

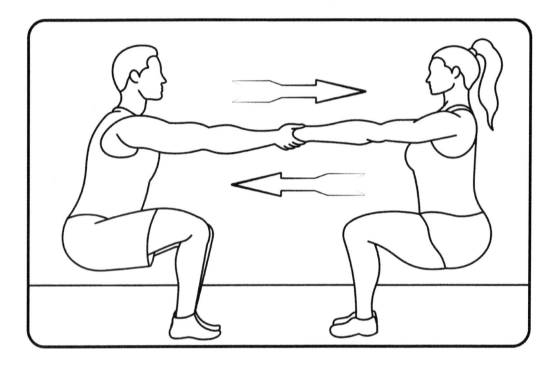

1.) Stand with your back to the wall, and then move about one pace away from it, facing your partner.

2.) Take your partner's right wrist with your right hand, and their left wrist with your left hand, crossing your arms. They should also be holding your wrists in their hands.

3.) Take a few moments to check that your bodies are in line with each other, with all of your joints facing their corresponding joints.

4.) Gradually begin to lean backwards and sit into a squat, keeping your spine upright as you go. Feel free to adjust your position (or your partner's position) until you find a comfortable arrangement.

5.) Squat down as far as your comfort allows, and then lift back up. Repeat this motion 5 times.

COOL-DOWN EXERCISES TO EASE
YOUR BODY INTO RECOVERY MODE

The cool-down is just as important as the warm-up for minimising the risk of injuries and preventing soreness. It gives your muscles an opportunity to relax and realise that the exercise period is over, and doing a proper cool-down should be a part of every exercise routine you do.

With that in mind, let's look at some cool-down exercises!

Exercise 1
Arm Pull

1.) Stand in a neutral position with your feet shoulder-width apart.

2.) Raise your arms straight in front of you, allowing your fingers to dangle towards the floor, but keeping your wrists in line with your elbows.

3.) Reach forwards, opening up your shoulder blades and drawing a deep breath in.

4.) As you exhale, consciously relax your shoulders, but keep your arms extended as much as possible, so that the muscles stretch.

5.) Pull your arms back in towards your body, letting your shoulder blades come back together.

6.) Relax your shoulders and drop your arms to your sides.

7.) Repeat this exercise 5 times.

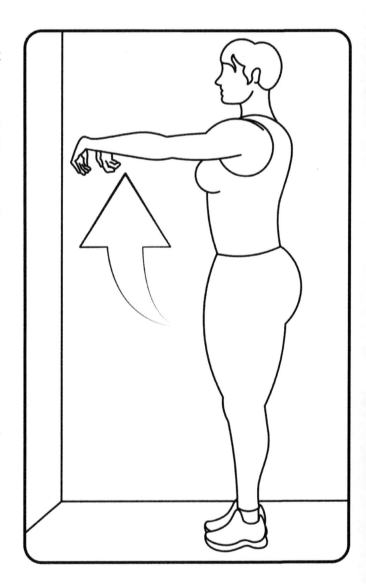

EXERCISE 2
SIDE LEG LIFTS

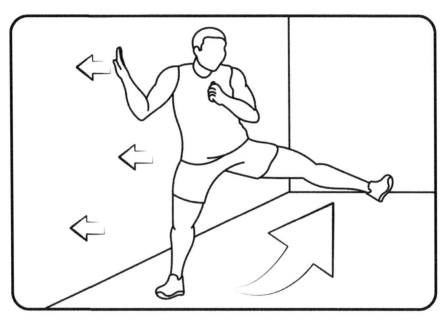

1.) Stand in a neutral position, with your right shoulder facing towards a wall. Place your hand on the wall for support.

2.) Lift your left foot off the floor and extend it out to the side of your body. You may find it helps to point your toes, as this makes it easier to keep your leg straight.

3.) Gradually lift your leg up to the side of your body as high as you comfortably can, and then hold it for a few seconds while you breathe deeply.

4.) Lower your leg and foot back to the floor, and then pick it up again. Repeat this 5 times.

5.) Turn so that your left shoulder faces the wall, and place your left hand on the wall for support.

6.) Repeat the exercise by lifting your right foot off the floor and extending your leg out to the side of your body as far as you comfortably can. Return it to the floor, and continue until you have completed 5 side lifts with your right leg.

EXERCISE 3
SEATED TOE-TAP

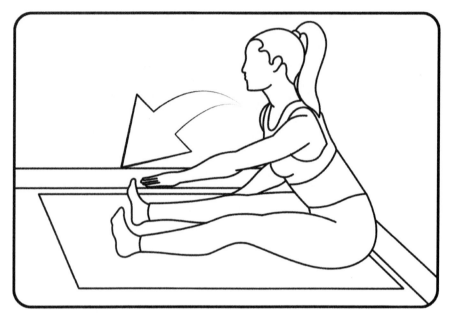

1.) Sit on the floor with your back against the wall. Line your joints up, and make sure most of your back is touching the wall. Your legs should be stretched out in front of you.

2.) Spread your legs out in front of you to around a hip's-width apart.

3.) Pull your abs tight, and then squeeze your lower back into the wall, holding your belly button taut.

4.) Reach your left hand towards your right foot, as though trying to tap your toes. If you can reach your toes, touch them, but don't go further than feels comfortable.

5.) Lean back against the wall, straighten up, and then do the same with your right hand reaching for your left foot.

6.) Repeat for about 45 seconds, alternating from side to side.

How to Personalise Your Wall Pilates Practise for Maximum Results

It's really important to remember, throughout your exercise journey, that you should be doing things at your own pace. Every individual develops at a different rate, and you should adapt the exercises in this book to fit a routine that suits you.

If you find exercises that are too hard for you, take a break and come back to them later. If you find exercises that are too easy for you, increase the number of repetitions, bump up the difficulty, or swap them for other exercises. This journey is unique to you, so never feel that you "should" be able to do this and your body is too slow or too weak; this is what training is about.

You should also take some time near the start of your journey to assess how different parts of your body feel. Identify areas of weakness – everyone has some, even people who exercise and stretch daily.

Remember that the things you do from day to day are likely to have an impact on what areas you need to work out. For example, if you frequently sit at a desk, you are likely to carry tension in your shoulders and neck. Other exercises that you do may also necessitate stretching in various ways, loosening up muscles and joints that have been made tight by your daily activities and workout routine.

Understanding what your weakest areas are will help you to maximise the benefits you get from doing Pilates, because it will help you to focus on these problem areas and address them effectively. This will make other aspects of your exercise more beneficial too, and may help you to bounce back more quickly after a workout session.

Personalisation isn't about deciding that you just don't like certain exercises, of course. Often, the exercises that feel uncomfortable and strenuous are the most important to try, because these are the ones that are exercising tight or weak muscles. Don't push beyond your comfort zone, but don't just skip over the exercises that are challenging in favour of doing things you already find easy.

Another aspect of personalising your Pilates journey is about knowing when your body needs to rest, and when you can't push harder. This is particularly crucial if you are watching videos online, and you want to imitate the instructor. Bear in mind that they do these exercises almost every day, and they will almost certainly have better flexibility and strength than you – so don't go beyond your comfort zone just because they do.

It can be surprising how hard different exercises are for different people. If you find a stretch is much more difficult than you anticipated, don't push hard just because you think it should be easy. Listen to your body, recognise when you are hitting a limit, and respect that limit. You can make a note to work on that area later, but don't go beyond what you are capable of.

Part of exercising safely involves paying attention to the cues your body is giving you and knowing when you can push a little further, but it often takes time to develop this understanding of your body's signs. Before you have it, err on the side of caution, and don't force something that feels uncomfortable.

Take your journey with wall Pilates as a journey just for yourself. Respect your limits, recognise and work on your weaknesses, and pay attention to what your body is saying. You'll get much better results this way!

How to make wall pilates
a daily habit with ease

Of course, a big part of making the most of Pilates is doing it very regularly. You don't have to make it through an hour's session every day, but you should be aiming to do at least a short session most days – and that can be challenging at first.

Exercising regularly takes a lot of determination and self-discipline. You might start out well, but soon find that you lose interest, and you start making excuses. The more you do this, the harder it is to make time, because it will always seem like an "extra" thing that you have to pack into an already busy day.

It's certainly challenging to make enough time for exercising sometimes, which is one of the reasons it's so important to simply make exercise part of your daily routine. With that in mind, let's look at a few tips.

Make A Time

When do you exercise? It's really important to have a specific time. This doesn't mean you can never exercise at any other time of day, but having some dedicated slots (or at least 1 dedicated slot) massively increases the chances that you will do the exercise you intend to do.

Think about when you are least likely to be interrupted by things like your phone, children, work, urgent messages, or chores such as cooking dinner. This might be first thing in the morning, during a lunch break, or an hour or two before bedtime. Whenever suits your routine best, make that your exercise slot, and try to always stick to it.

Bear in mind that it doesn't need to be a long slot – two or even three short slots will also be fine! Just fit it in whenever you can.

You should supplement this technique by setting a reminder on your phone, a watch, or something else, especially when you first start exercising. Having a physical reminder can be key to making sure that you remember, and that you actually get up and do it – so don't underestimate the value of this.

MAKE IT EASY

You don't need a lot of equipment or setup for wall Pilates, which is one of the things that makes it so accessible, but it's still worth thinking about ways in which you can make it as easy as possible to exercise.

For example, making sure you have a clear space around the wall you're going to use, and getting your exercise clothes ready is a good start. If you have to tidy your whole living room before you can exercise, you're not likely to do it, so remember to set your space up in advance!

SET NEW GOALS

Often, when you start exercising, you have lots of goals in mind and you're very excited to get started. However, as you progress and hit those goals, you may find that your motivation starts to diminish, and you lose interest.

You can counteract this by setting yourself lots of ongoing, mini goals. This will help you to feel like you are achieving and progressing, rather than stagnating. Having multiple small goals ensures you get a good sense of achievement and satisfaction, and tends to be easier to keep up than having just a few big goals.

Remember to reward yourself when you achieve a goal, too, because this will keep you motivated and energised.

DON'T GIVE UP IF YOU MISS A SESSION

Some people feel that as soon as they miss a workout session, they might as well give up on exercising – but that's something you should be careful to avoid. Exercise isn't all or nothing; it's about doing the best you can. If you miss a session, simply resume your next session as soon as you can.

That's true no matter how many sessions you have missed; you can always get back to it! Don't just tell yourself "tomorrow" constantly; simply jump back in!

WALL PILATES
FAQs

Q: WHO INVENTED PILATES?

A: Pilates was developed in the 1920s by a man named Joseph Pilates. Joseph Pilates had suffered from ill health as a child, and took a great interest in fitness techniques that would allow him to build up his physical and mental strength. He spent a long time practising many different forms of exercise, combining both Western and Eastern ideas to create the exercise that has become so popular today.

Q: HOW LONG SHOULD A PILATES SESSION BE?

A: Although it is a low-impact exercise that depends upon controlled movements, a good Pilates workout can increase your heart rate and improve your cardiovascular health. However, it often takes a while to work up to this point, and it may not be easy, so if your doctor has recommended cardiovascular exercise, look at other forms of working out.

Q: IS PILATES A WHOLE-BODY WORKOUT?

A: Yes, when done correctly, Pilates gives you a full-body workout. It tones your legs, abdominal muscles, arms, back, shoulders, and more.

Of course, if you only focus on one area, you won't get much of a workout for other muscle groups, but it's very easy to create balanced exercise plans with a Pilates workout, which is one of the reasons this has become a popular form of exercise.

WALL PILATES
FAQs

Q: WHY IS PILATES DIFFERENT FROM OTHER KINDS OF EXERCISE?

A: All exercises are unique, but one of the main things that sets Pilates apart from other exercises is that it's low impact. That means you're not likely to hurt yourself by doing it (provided you do it correctly), making it a safe option for individuals everywhere – even those dealing with physical impairments.

Furthermore, it works your body out in symmetrical, even ways that feel great. Pilates does have a lot in common with exercises like yoga, but it tends to use more resistance, and can provide a more intense workout as a result.

Q: HOW OFTEN CAN YOU DO PILATES?

A: Again, this depends on you to an extent, but most people can safely do Pilates every day if they aren't pushing too hard. It's a relatively gentle form of exercise. Joseph Pilates recommended that individuals do it three times a week, and many people aim to do it every other day.

Remember the importance of not overtraining, and be sensible when you create your exercise routine. On the whole, it's better to err on the side of doing too little, rather than too much!

Glossary and Additional Resources

Glossary

It may help to have a list of the terms that are commonly used in the Pilates world. A few have appeared in this book (defined where appropriate), and will reappear here for the sake of clarity and completeness. Use this glossary to enhance your understanding of the Pilates world and any other resources you may be using that contain these terms.

Abduction: Your shoulder blades move away from the spine

Adduction: Your shoulder blades move towards the spine

Anterior: Your front side (or a movement to the front)

Centring: Strengthening the centre of your body, the powerhouse, while exercising

C-Curve: Your spine is rounded and even, like a capital C, with your body curved forwards

Dorsiflexion: A flexed foot

Eccentric Muscle Action: the muscle lengthening and working

Extension: A movement that increases the angle of your joints (straightening them)

Flexion: Rounding

Foot Walk: Walking on the balls of your feet, with your heels clear of the ground

Intercostal Muscles: The muscles found between your ribs that help you to breathe

Lateral: To the side (either referring to body parts or to a movement to the side)

Midline: A straight line running from the top of your head to your feet

Neutral Pelvis: When your pelvis is held level, with the hip bones in line with each other and with the pubic bone

Parallel Stance: A position where your knees, legs, and feet are aligned beneath your hips

GLOSSARY AND
ADDITIONAL RESOURCES
GLOSSARY

Pilates Stance or the Pilates V: A position where you are standing in alignment, except for your feet. Your heels should touch, while your toes are turned out from each other at a 45-degree angle, a little like a ballet dancer standing in turnout position.

Posterior: The back of the body (either referring to body parts or a movement backwards)

Powerhouse: The region from the bottom of your ribs to the line of your hips. This includes your pelvic floor, your hip muscles, your glutes, your abs, and your lower back muscles, and it's a key aspect of Pilates

Scoop Abs: Pulling your ab muscles inwards to support your back

Supine: Lying on the floor flat on your back

ADDITIONAL RESOURCES

This book has aimed to provide a comprehensive, in-depth, and useful guide to doing wall Pilates for beginners, with some intermediate and even advanced exercises thrown in. However, there are plenty more resources that you can tap into if you are interested in learning even more about Pilates.

There are other books available, but you might find that YouTube videos make an excellent supplement. One of the best ways to practise wall Pilates, though, is to join a proper class. There are lots available and this can be an excellent option for meeting new people, getting real-time feedback about your technique, and holding yourself accountable.

If you don't have a local class, consider joining some online sessions. There are again many great options, and you will learn a lot from them.

Index

Printed in Great Britain
by Amazon